QI GONG EXERCISES FOR BEGINNERS

Elevate Mind And Body, Essential Qi Gong Exercises For Vitality, Health, Holistic Wellness And Inner Balance

LAMBERT FETTERMAN

DISCLAIMER

The content in this book is offered only for general informative purposes. While every effort has been taken to guarantee the content's accuracy and completeness, the author and publisher accept no responsibility for any mistakes or omissions, or for the results of using the information given herein. The methods, recommendations, and directions in this book are not guaranteed to be appropriate for every person, and readers should exercise caution and seek professional counsel if required before undertaking any of the projects or techniques detailed in this book.

Table of Contents

INTRODUCTION

Qi Gong, an ancient Chinese practice, has several physical and mental health advantages. Its presentation enables newcomers to grasp its core and ideas, signaling the start of a path toward holistic health.

Exploring Qi Gong: A Brief Overview

Qi Gong, pronounced "chee-gong," is a practice that consists of gentle movements, breathing exercises, and concentrated intentions that encourage the flow of Qi (vital life energy) throughout the body. This practice, based on Traditional Chinese Medicine (TCM), strives to harmonize the body, mind, and spirit, promoting balance and vigor.

Understanding The Principles Behind Qi Gong

Several essential ideas underpin Qi Gong. The idea of Qi, the energy thought to move through the body via particular paths known as meridians, is central to all of these. Qi Gong practitioners strive to improve the smooth flow of Qi to retain health and avoid sickness. This flow is affected by the three pillars of Qi Gong practice: mind, breath, and movement.

Breathing deeply and deliberately is essential to Qi Gong, allowing for the intake of new Qi and the discharge of stagnant energy. Mindful movement, especially slow and deliberate activities, enhances Qi flow, promoting physical flexibility and strength while simultaneously soothing the mind. Intention and imagination boost the benefits of Qi Gong even further, enabling practitioners to focus their Qi on particular locations for healing and balance.

The introduction to Qi Gong prepares novices by providing an overview of the practice's deep ideas and its capacity to balance the body, mind, and spirit.

CHAPTER 1

The Fundamentals Of Qi Gong

Origins And History Of Qi Gong

Qi Gong is an ancient Chinese practice that is strongly entrenched in traditional Chinese medicine, martial arts, and philosophy. It has a long history, emerging from a combination of spiritual, physical, and contemplative activities. Qi Gong began with the goal of developing life force energy ('Qi') for health, vigor, and self-defense.

Key Concepts: Qi, Yin And Yang, Five Elements

• Qi: A vital life force or energy that passes through the body, 'Qi' is central to Qi Gong. Qi Gong activities are designed to regulate, balance, and improve the flow of Qi for improved health and well-being.

• Yin and Yang: Qi Gong is an embodiment of the Yin-Yang philosophy, which emphasizes the balance and harmony of opposing energies. It assists practitioners in achieving mental, bodily, and energy balance.

• Five Elements Theory: The notion of the Five Elements (Wood, Fire, Earth, Metal, Water) signifying interrelated energies has impacted Qi Gong. Practitioners connect workouts and motions with these factors to achieve bodily balance and harmony.

Benefits Of Practicing Qi Gong

Qi Gong has several advantages:

• Improves health by increasing flexibility, muscular strength, circulation, and immune system function.

• Stress Reduction: Aids in relaxation, calming the mind, and stress relief.

• Energy Cultivation: Promotes vitality and mental clarity by cultivating and balancing Qi.

• Mind-Body Connection: Strengthens the bond between the mind, body, and spirit, promoting overall well-being.

The gentle, flowing movements of Qi Gong, combined with breathwork and mindfulness, make it suitable for beginners seeking physical, mental, and spiritual well-being.

CHAPTER 2

Breathing Techniques In Qi Gong

Breathing practices are crucial in Qi Gong, providing as the basis for practice. They play a critical role in directing the flow of Qi (vital energy) throughout the body. Understanding and mastering different breathing patterns has a huge influence on the efficacy of Qi Gong workouts.

Importance Of Breath In Qi Gong Exercises

Qi Gong emphasizes the coordination of breath and movement. Proper breathing patterns promote a smooth flow of Qi, promoting relaxation, focus, and energy cultivation. To regulate energy flow, improve concentration, and aid in relaxation, inhalation, and exhalation techniques are combined with specific movements.

Different Breathing Patterns And Their Effects

1. Qi Gong encourages abdominal breathing (diaphragmatic breathing), in which the diaphragm contracts and expands, allowing for deeper inhalations. This technique promotes relaxation, reduces stress, and helps the body oxygenate.

2. Natural Breathing: Qi Gong emphasizes natural breathing, which allows the breath to flow naturally and without effort. It aids

practitioners in attaining a relaxed and meditative state.

3. Reverse Breathing entails expanding the abdomen while inhaling and contracting it while exhaling. Reverse breathing increases strength and focus during Qi Gong exercises by stimulating energy circulation.

4. Coordinated Breathing: Coordinating inhalation and exhalation with transitions in Qi Gong exercises helps unify body and mind, optimizing energy flow.

Learning Diaphragmatic Breathing

The foundation of Qi Gong's breathwork is diaphragmatic breathing, also known as abdominal or deep breathing. To put this technique into practice, do the following:

• Posture: Maintain a relaxed, upright posture while standing or sitting comfortably.

• Hand placement: Gently place your hands on your lower abdomen, near the navel.

• Inhalation: Breathe slowly and deeply through your nose, letting your abdomen rise. Feel the lower belly expand, allowing air to fill the lungs.

• Exhalation: Slowly exhale through the mouth or nose, allowing the abdomen to naturally fall. With each exhalation, feel the tension release and let go of any stress or negativity.

• Mindful Focus: While breathing, concentrate on the rhythm of your breath, the sensation of your abdomen rising and falling, and the calming effect it has.

Practicing and mastering various Qi Gong breathing techniques builds a solid foundation for harnessing Qi, improving relaxation, and promoting overall well-being. Beyond physical exercise, these techniques can be incorporated into daily routines to reap the many benefits of Qi Gong.

CHAPTER 3

Basic Qi Gong Movements

Qi Gong exercises, which emphasize the flow of energy or "Qi" throughout the body, are deeply rooted in Chinese culture. These exercises have numerous advantages for both physical and mental health. Let's take a closer look at Chapter 3: Basic Qi Gong Movements to better understand these gentle yet powerful exercises.

Gentle Warm-Up Exercises

To prepare the body and mind for practice, Qi Gong frequently begins with gentle warm-up exercises. Joint rotations, gentle stretches, and soft movements designed to increase circulation, loosen muscles, and promote relaxation may be included. Warm-ups are necessary to ease into the more focused Qi Gong postures and movements.

Stances And Postures For Qi Gong

Qi Gong is all about posture. Practitioners learn various stances and positions to help Qi flow smoothly. A stable stance is essential for rooting oneself to the ground. Beginners usually begin with simple postures like Wu Ji (standing meditation), concentrating on alignment, relaxation, and proper breathing while maintaining a centered posture.

Exploring Simple Qi Gong Forms

Qi Gong forms are a series of flowing, coordinated movements that are often inspired by nature or animals. These forms are typically simple for beginners, allowing them to focus on the fundamental principles of Qi Gong, such as relaxation, breath control, and body alignment.

These simple forms may include gentle arm movements, waist rotations, and weight shifts from one leg to the other, promoting coordination and balance while instilling inner calm. Slow, deliberate movements allow practitioners to synchronize their breath and movement, promoting a meditative state.

Beginners gradually develop an understanding of how energy flows within their bodies and learn to harness this energy for health and vitality by focusing on these basic Qi Gong movements.

Each of these fundamental exercises lays the groundwork for more advanced Qi Gong practices, guiding beginners toward improved physical balance, mental clarity, and a stronger connection to their inner energy. As practitioners progress, they can explore more complex forms and variations, but starting with the fundamentals is critical for establishing a solid foundation in Qi Gong's practice.

CHAPTER 4

Building Qi Awareness

Sensing And Cultivating Qi Flow

Understanding and sensing Qi, the vital life force energy, is essential in Qi Gong's practice. Beginners learn to perceive Qi flow within their bodies. Through gentle movements, breathwork, and focused attention, practitioners gradually develop sensitivity to the subtle energies circulating within. Techniques involve mindful awareness of sensations like warmth, tingling, or pulsations while performing Qi Gong exercises.

Practitioners also learn to guide and enhance Qi flow through mental focus and intention.

Visualization Techniques In Qi Gong

Visualization plays a pivotal role in Qi Gong's practice. It involves mentally directing Qi to specific areas or pathways within the body. Beginners engage in guided imagery, picturing Qi as a radiant light or flowing streams circulating through the body's energy channels (meridians). Visualization aids in fostering Qi awareness, promoting relaxation, and aligning the mind-body connection.

Developing Mindfulness And Concentration

Qi Gong cultivates a meditative state, fostering mindfulness and concentration. Beginners practice being fully present in the moment, focusing attention on breath, movement, and the flow of Qi.

Through repetitive movements and controlled breathing, practitioners enhance concentration, quieting the mind's distractions. This heightened awareness not only deepens the Qi Gong practice but also extends the benefits into daily life.

Progression In Qi Awareness

As beginners progress, their Qi awareness evolves. They refine their ability to sense subtle energy movements and patterns. The practice helps in recognizing how Qi responds to thoughts, emotions, and physical movements. Advanced practitioners can guide and manipulate Qi intentionally, benefiting overall health and wellness.

CHAPTER 5

Qi Gong For Relaxation And Stress Relief

Relaxation Techniques In Qi Gong

Qi Gong exercises often focus on slow, deliberate movements combined with intentional breathing. These gentle movements encourage relaxation by releasing tension held in the body.

The emphasis on smooth, flowing motions and controlled breathing helps calm the nervous system, allowing the body to enter a state of relaxation.

Stress Reduction Practices

One of the primary purposes of Qi Gong is to alleviate stress. Through its various movements and breath work, Qi Gong can effectively reduce stress levels. By promoting relaxation and improving the body's response to stress, practitioners experience reduced anxiety and an increased sense of calm.

Qi Gong's emphasis on mindfulness and being present at the moment encourages a break from daily stressors. As individuals focus on their movements and breath, it creates a meditative state that can counteract the effects of stress.

Using Qi Gong For Mental Clarity And Emotional Balance

In addition to physical relaxation, Qi Gong helps foster mental clarity and emotional balance. The slow, intentional movements allow individuals to connect with their inner selves, fostering a sense of harmony and emotional stability.

Regular practice of Qi Gong can enhance mental focus and clarity. By calming the mind and reducing mental chatter, practitioners often experience improved concentration and mental acuity in their daily lives.

Furthermore, Qi Gong's emphasis on balancing the body's energy can help regulate emotions. By harmonizing the flow of Qi, practitioners often report feeling emotionally balanced, more centered, and better equipped to handle life's challenges.

CHAPTER 6

Balancing Qi: Exercises For Harmony

Balancing Yin And Yang Energies

In Qi Gong, the principles of Yin and Yang serve as fundamental concepts for achieving harmony and balance within the body. Yin represents the receptive, nurturing, and passive aspects, while Yang embodies the active, dynamic, and expressive qualities. Through specific movements and breathing techniques, practitioners aim to harmonize and balance these opposing energies, fostering equilibrium for overall well-being.

Working With The Five Elements

The Five Elements Theory—Wood, Fire, Earth, Metal, and Water—is deeply integrated into Qi Gong's practice. Each element corresponds to specific organs, emotions, seasons, and energy patterns within the body. Qi Gong exercises are designed to activate and balance these elements, ensuring smooth energy flow and fostering harmony between the body, mind, and environment.

Harmonizing Qi Through Movement And Stillness

Qi Gong emphasizes both movement-based exercises and meditative stillness to harmonize Qi. Dynamic movements help circulate and balance energy throughout the body, while static postures or meditation practices aid in grounding and internalizing Qi. By alternating between active and passive exercises, practitioners attain a balanced state of energy flow, promoting harmony and vitality.

Importance of Harmonizing Qi for Health and Well-being

Achieving harmony in Qi is believed to promote holistic health—physically, mentally, and emotionally. When Qi flows smoothly and harmoniously through the body's meridians, it supports the optimal functioning of organs, enhances mental clarity, reduces stress, and fosters emotional stability. Balancing Qi is considered essential for maintaining overall well-being and preventing illness.

CHAPTER 7

Qi Gong For Health And Healing

Strengthening The Immune System Through Qi Gong

Qi Gong exercises are renowned for their potential to boost the immune system. Regular practice may enhance the body's overall resilience against illnesses by improving circulation, reducing stress hormones, and promoting relaxation. Qi Gong's focus on deep breathing and gentle movements can stimulate the lymphatic system, facilitating the body's natural defense mechanisms.

Addressing Common Health Issues With Qi Gong

Qi Gong is often used to manage and alleviate various health conditions. It's employed as a complementary approach alongside conventional medicine to aid in conditions like chronic pain, hypertension, anxiety, and even chronic illnesses like asthma or arthritis. The slow, deliberate movements, combined with focused breathing and mental relaxation, can contribute to pain reduction and stress relief, offering a holistic approach to wellness.

Qi Gong As Complementary Therapy

In healthcare settings, Qi Gong is increasingly recognized as a complementary therapy. Many individuals integrate Qi Gong into their treatment plans, finding it supportive in managing symptoms and improving overall health. It's used alongside other treatments, such as physical therapy or medication, to address different aspects of health—physical, mental, and emotional.

Practicing Qi Gong regularly under the guidance of a qualified instructor might help individuals better manage chronic conditions, enhance their overall health, and improve their quality of life.

CHAPTER 8

Developing Strength And Flexibility

Qi Gong, an ancient practice originating from China, offers numerous benefits for both physical and mental well-being. Let's delve into Chapter 8, focusing on how Qi Gong aids in developing strength, flexibility, and endurance.

Enhancing Physical Strength With Qi Gong

Qi Gong exercises involve various postures, stances, and movements that engage different muscle groups in the body. While the movements might seem gentle, they can gradually enhance overall physical strength.

By practicing Qi Gong regularly, individuals often notice improvements in muscle tone and strength, particularly in the legs, core, and back muscles.

The slow and controlled nature of Qi Gong's movements requires maintaining muscle tension and stability, contributing to muscle strength development. Additionally, some Qi Gong forms involve holding specific postures or performing repetitive movements, which act as isometric exercises, effectively engaging and strengthening muscles without the need for heavy lifting or strain.

Improving Flexibility And Range Of Motion

Flexibility is a crucial aspect of fitness that Qi Gong helps enhance. The flowing, gentle movements in Qi Gong exercises involve stretching and elongating various muscle groups, promoting flexibility throughout the body. With regular practice, individuals experience increased joint flexibility and improved range of motion, which can aid in preventing injuries and relieving stiffness.

Qi Gong emphasizes movements that encourage joint mobility, such as gentle twists, rotations, and circular motions, fostering suppleness and elasticity in muscles and connective tissues. This can be especially beneficial for individuals with sedentary lifestyles or those experiencing tightness due to stress or prolonged sitting.

Qi Gong For Muscular Endurance

Muscular endurance refers to the ability of muscles to perform tasks repeatedly without fatigue. Qi Gong's slow, continuous movements challenge muscles to sustain effort over an extended period. By incorporating controlled breathing and rhythmic movements, Qi Gong exercises build endurance gradually.

Practicing Qi Gong forms that involve holding postures or performing sequences of movements for extended durations strengthens muscles and improves their endurance. As the body becomes accustomed to sustaining these postures, individuals may notice increased stamina and reduced muscular fatigue in daily activities.

In summary, Qi Gong offers a holistic approach to physical fitness, enhancing strength, flexibility, and muscular endurance through its gentle yet purposeful movements. Incorporating Qi Gong into a regular exercise routine can contribute significantly to overall physical health and well-being.

CHAPTER 9

Qi Gong For Mind-Body Connection

Qi Gong's essence lies in nurturing the mind-body connection, fostering harmony between mental and physical well-being.

Integrating Mindfulness And Meditation In Qi Gong

Qi Gong emphasizes mindfulness, training practitioners to be present in the moment. Through slow, deliberate movements and concentrated breathing, people create a heightened awareness of their bodies, minds, and environment. This exercise develops a contemplative state, soothing the mind and lowering tension.

Embracing Mind-Body Harmony

By coordinating movements with breath and concentrating the attention on these acts, Qi Gong promotes a seamless connection between body and mind. Practitioners typically feel a sense of harmony and balance, boosting their general well-being.

Cultivating Emotional Well-Being

Qi Gong's gentle, regular motions and regulated breathing help ease emotional tension. Regular practice may help regulate emotions, decrease anxiety, and increase emotional stability.

The contemplative part of Qi Gong assists in developing mental clarity and cultivating a positive view of life.

CHAPTER 10

Incorporating Qi Gong Into Daily Life

Qi Gong isn't only about the time spent training; it's about incorporating its concepts throughout daily life for continuing benefits.

Establishing A Regular Practice Routine

Building a steady Qi Gong practice doesn't necessarily imply extended hours every day. Even short, frequent sessions may bring considerable advantages. Start gently, maybe 10 to 15 minutes a day, and gradually raise the length as you get comfortable. Find a time that works best for you, whether it's early morning, during a break at work, or in the evening before bed.

Applying Qi Gong Principles Beyond Exercises

Qi Gong's concepts extend well beyond the physical motions. During practice, you will learn mindfulness, breathing methods, and energy cultivation techniques that you may use throughout the day. Mindful breathing may assist in reducing stress, and centering activities can help restore attention amid hectic schedules.

Implementing Qi Gong In Various Aspects Of Life

Qi Gong concepts may be used in a variety of activities. While walking, sitting, or even working at a desk, include slow, deliberate motions and aware breathing. While standing in line or stuck in traffic, practicing Qi Gong exercises quietly helps improve posture and energy flow.

By incorporating Qi Gong into your everyday life, you may reap its advantages outside of practice sessions. You practice mindfulness, decrease stress, and improve your general well-being by cultivating a harmonious connection between mind, body, and spirit in all aspects of life. Remember that the purpose is to live in a manner that represents the core of Qi Gong, not only to do exercises.

Conclusion

Beginning your Qi Gong adventure will expose you to a world of deep mind-body activities. You've learned about the core ideas, exercises, and potential changes that Qi Gong has to offer. As you finish this beginner's guide, it's important to reflect on the road you've taken and the opportunities ahead.

Accept The Experience

Qi Gong is more than just a set of exercises; it is a way of life that promotes harmony and balance. Your investigation has allowed you to experience the essence of Qi cultivation, combining movement and awareness, and promoting health and vitality.

Journey Continued

Remember that Qi Gong's mastery is a continual practice. The prerequisites to realizing its full potential are consistency and perseverance. The depth of your knowledge will deepen as you continue, exposing new levels of energy cultivation and inner serenity.

Integration Into Daily Life

The ideas and practices taught are not limited to practice sessions. Accept the incorporation of Qi Gong into your everyday life. The advantages of cultivating awareness during boring chores, employing breathing methods in difficult times, or incorporating Qi Gong concepts into your relationships extend beyond the practice mat.

Community And Help

Exploring Qi Gong introduces you to new communities and resources. Engage with other practitioners, get advice from instructors, and keep learning. Collective knowledge and shared experiences might help you get a better understanding and drive you to practice.

Thank you and acknowledgement

Take a minute to recognize your dedication and discipline on this trip. Your devotion to learning about Qi Gong's concepts and exercises is admirable.

Recognize your progress, no matter how tiny, since it is the cornerstone of a huge shift.

Looking Ahead

Consider this guide to be a stepping stone rather than a goal. Accept the idea of further development and refinement. The gift of Qi Gong is its ageless character, which invites you to explore its depths and experience its tremendous impacts on an ongoing basis.

Finally, may your Qi Gong journey bring you balance, tranquillity, and well-being, directing you on a road to holistic health and self-awareness.

THE END

61